The Grapefruit
And
Apple Cider Vinegar
Combo Diet

Randall Earl Dunford

Magni Group, Inc.

Disclaimer

The information presented in this publication is designed to inform and educate the reader with the view to making intelligent choices in regard to a healthy life-style. None of the material included within is intended to replace the advice of your physician, especially in respect to the very young, the weak elderly, those taking medications, diabetics, or anyone with a serious health condition. Neither the author or the publisher assumes any responsibility or liability for the judgments or decisions any reader might reach as a result of reading this volume. Please remember, too, that no one can expect to receive the full benefits from grapefruit and apple cider vinegar if a responsible life-style is not maintained.

Contents

Introduction

The word "loss" almost always holds negative implications. We become concerned when we misplace our car keys. We feel dejected when our favorite team loses a game. Likewise, we may shudder at the very thought of a stock market heading south. But there is one instance in which the concept of loss more often than not holds the fragrance of victory: when it is applied to the weight of the human body.

The reality of that victory, however, has been elusive to most. Excess weight is a lingering, formidable enemy of far too many in the world today. It is, in fact, a mounting problem. In the past 10 years, the incidence of obesity in adults has increased from one in four to one in three, while adolescent obesity since 1980 has grown by a staggering 40%!

Obesity, it appears, is becoming our master. It's a burden we must carry around every waking moment. Some of us have tried everything short of jumping off a bridge to achieve the weight we desire. If cutting back on calories doesn't do the trick, we may decide fasting is the answer. Failing this, we might embark on a heavy exercise program. In desperation, some of us even give drugs a whirl. In the end, however, failure usually reigns.

This book is directed toward those seeking an effective and permanent solution to this problem. Its centerpiece involves the utilization of a well-known citrus fruit, the grapefruit, coupled with variations of an enduring, well-proven application made prominent by Dr. D. C. Jarvis, a renown Vermont physician—the regular use of a teaspoonful of apple cider vinegar in a glass of water.

We, however, are going to considerably expand this basic concept by incorporating some creative meals and homemade beverages into a healthy, nourishing diet designed to please the palate. You will even have your choice of how much weight you want to lose by deciding how much time you are willing to invest in your diet. There will be three options: The Express Diet (a three-day plan), the Intermediate Diet (a ten-day plan) and the Extended Diet (a thirty-day plan). And you won't ever have to skip a meal.

By putting one of these diets to work, and investing a modest amount of time each day for simple exercise, you will soon discover how easy it can be to succeed in losing weight and keeping it off once and for all. Ready? Well turn the page and let's get started.

Part 1

Introducing the Players

Chapter 1

A Dynamic Duo

We've heard much in recent times about how effective apple cider vinegar can be in regard to helping one shed those unwanted pounds. But there is another highly nutritious food known as the grapefruit, which plays an equally big role in this respect. Combine the two and what do you have? One whale of a powerful formula beautifully designed for achieving a trim figure.

A Chemical Marriage Made in Heaven

What makes it work so well? It largely concerns the ability of the apple cider vinegar to aid in suppressing the appetite as well as to help regulate the metabolism, a process that's expedited by the grapefruit, which, among other attributes, possesses the ability to enhance the absorption of all that the body ingests—including, of course, the cider vinegar itself. In fact, the grapefruit is so efficient at this, that that's the reason a caution is out for those taking certain medications who desire to eat this fruit. (Anyone, therefore, who is on medication should check with his or her physician before embarking on the grapefruit and apple cider vinegar combo diet.)

It's only fitting that these two major players are such an excellent choice when it comes to weight control because they both contain virtually no fat or sodium. What's more, both grapefruit and apple cider vinegar are completely natural and include important vitamins and minerals essential for a healthy life.

Incorporating Grapefruit and Apple Cider Vinegar Into the Diet

At this stage, you might be inclined to think that a grapefruit and apple cider vinegar diet would get pretty darn boring in a hurry. You may well visualize eating a grapefruit or two at most every meal along with skimpy portions of a few other foods from a limited menu and washing it all down with a teaspoonful of apple cider vinegar in a glass of water. But it's surprisingly easy to put into action this powerful combination in ways which are creative as well as effective. Apple cider vinegar can be incorporated into more appetizing dishes than you may realize. It can be mixed in sauces and dressings and there are numerous entrees which can use it in their recipes. And in many cases the helpings don't even have to be small. Grapefruit juice as well as the vinegar can be put to work in a wide range of appealing beverages which will enhance the enjoyment of your meals.

Before we jump headlong into a diet, however, let's get a better idea of just how this potent pair can help you to lose those nagging extra pounds.

Caution For Those On Medication

Please remember that anyone taking medication absolutely must check with his or her physician before embarking on the grapefruit and apple cider vinegar combo diet because grapefruit may intensify the effect of the dosage to harmful levels. There might be a lesson here for medical science. Why could this knowledge not be applied toward finding ways to utilize the properties of the grapefruit for medications so that smaller dosages will work more efficiently?

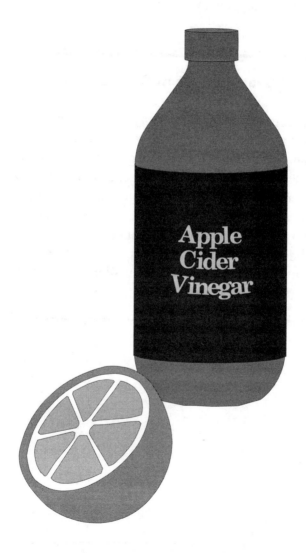

Chapter 2

The Glorious Grapefruit

The grapefruit (citrus paradisi) is a juicy lemon-yellow-colored fruit with a distinctive, mildly acid flavor. Its size averages roughly twice as large as a medium-sized orange, and in fact represents the largest member of the citrus family. Red- or pink-pulp grapefruits are normally larger, sweeter and less acidic than their white-pulp cousin and can often be identified by a slight pinkish hue in their yellow skin. The grapefruit earned its name because of the fact that it grows in clusters, somewhat reminiscent of grapes. This fruit is still widely accepted today, primarily as a breakfast food.

During the middle of the twentieth century, the grapefruit became a hot item for those who wanted to lose weight. It's popularity in this regard began to diminish, however, in the wake of many gimmick diets that promised swift success with minimal effort. That's a pity because this refreshing citrus fruit can play an important role in helping one to shed those pesky pounds.

What's in a Grapefruit?

What exactly makes a grapefruit tick? Let's chemically dissect one and see. A listing of some of its properties will help us more fully determine how significant it is in helping one to lose weight.

Among other constituents, a typical ½ medium grapefruit contains 160 milligrams of potassium, 1.3 grams of dietary fiber (including the kind known as pectin), and 10 grams of carbohydrates, as well as 0.8 grams of protein that include several important amino acids (the building blocks of protein), and vitamin A (largely in the form of beta carotene), vitamin C (ascorbic acid), and bioflavonoids, not to mention water—all packed into just 37 calories. In fact, as a source of vitamin C, the grapefruit is exceeded only by the orange and lemon, providing 100% of the daily recommended allowance.

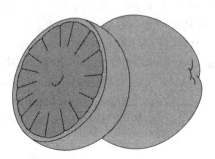

A grapefruit contains 100% of the daily recommended allowance of vitamin C.

**Some of the Healthful Ingredients
in a Typical Grapefruit**

Serving size ½ medium red or white

- Potassium: 160 milligrams
- Fiber: 1.3 grams
- Carbohydrates: 10 grams
- Protein: 0.8 grams
- Vitamin C: 40 milligrams
- Vitamin A:*   12 International Units (white)
                     153 International Units (red)

*Grapefruit (as with any other fruit or vegetable) does not actually *contain* vitamin A. More accurately, it contains many carotenes such as alpha carotene and beta carotene (also known as pro-vitamin A), which is, in a sense, an incomplete version of the vitamin. The human body converts this into the full-blown vitamin A after it is consumed.

The Importance of Grapefruit Components

Just how important are these components? For one thing, grapefruits contain so much water and fiber that they will fill one up quickly. Fiber produces a more filling effect because it contributes texture to the product, while water's ability in this regard is easy enough to understand.

This is undoubtedly the most obvious factor when considering weight control.

Another ingredient important in the pound-shedding battle involves one of the amino acids that make up the protein content. Of the three occurring naturally in grapefruit (tryptophan, lysine, and methionine), the one that especially concerns us is tryptophan. Those who are short on tryptophan have a tendency to crave sweets. Therefore, it plays a significant role in helping one to put down the sweet snacks, which all too often contain much fat.

Potassium also turns out to be a notable factor because it reacts in the body the opposite way to that of sodium. Sodium sucks water into the blood, thereby allowing the body to retain more liquid and therefore more weight. Potassium, on the other hand, helps maintain the fluid balance in the body's cells by transporting water to the kidneys to be excreted.

The carbohydrates, found in healthy foods such as the grapefruit, are also important because they break down sugars in the body which release insulin. This insulin manufactures hormones that somewhat step up the metabolic rate. As the metabolism increases, more calories are in turn burned off.

Other constituents worthy of note are bioflavonoids (also referred to as vitamin P), compounds which are responsible for the color of grapefruit. Along with vitamin C, bioflavonoids help activate the accumulation of fat-freeing hormones and enzymes.

In addition to all of this, because of the grapefruit's capacity to enhance the absorption of all that the human system takes in, the body is able to more efficiently utilize all the food it receives, therefore helping one to remain satisfied longer so he or she does not feel hungry as soon. In other words, it helps to put off the appetite.

Other Health Benefits of the Grapefruit

Grapefruit is not only excellent in helping one lose weight, it is an extremely healthy food in many ways. According to a list compiled by the Center for Science in the Public Interest (a privately funded consumer health advocacy organization), the grapefruit is the fifth most nutritious fruit behind cantaloupes, watermelon, oranges, and strawberries.

The vitamin A is important in maintaining good vision and helps keep the respiratory passages functioning normally. It also prevents skin diseases. Vitamin C, among other things, is essential for the production of new cells and tissues. It can also lessen the severity of colds and flu. Recent studies suggest that it might even help prevent gastric and esophageal cancer.

Some of the bioflavonoids help to prevent the spread of malignant cells within the body. Working in concert with vitamin C, bioflavonoids also have antiviral properties, promote healthy capillaries, and reduce problems such as gum bleeding. In fact, the benefits of vitamin C are boosted up to twenty times because of these bioflavonoids.

The pectin, the soluble fiber located in the pulpy membranes that separate the individual sections of the grapefruit, can also help lower blood cholesterol levels. Grapefruit pectin, in fact, turns out to be the most effective at this job. This process is made even more efficient by the vitamin C.

Grapefruit also contains compounds known as terpenes. These terpenes help to produce enzymes that limit the production of cholesterol and disable carcinogens. As a result, the arteries are protected from disease and risk of cancer is lowered, especially in regard to the stomach and pancreas.

Grapefruit, also contains coumarins. These substances serve as natural blood thinners, which it is suspected may help prevent blood clots, thereby reducing the chance of heart disease and stroke.

Also, another compound called galacturonic acid, found only in grapefruit, is believed to add a unique therapeutic benefit. It appears to dislodge the accumulation of fatty plaque in arteries and clear it away.

Another substance called lycopene (a relative of beta carotene) is found in red grapefruit. It is thought to prevent cancer of the prostate, colon, bladder, cervix, and lung.

Much more can be said about the health benefits of grapefruit. It also cleans the intestines and strengthens the immune system. In addition, it stimulates the liver and helps with elimination.

How To Eat A Grapefruit

Using a spoon to pull out the flesh between each section is not the best technique for eating a grapefruit. This way, one gets little more than the juice. To derive maximum benefit from this fruit, one should peel it like an orange and consume the slices.

Some even claim a nightly grapefruit will help you sleep. National health food practitioners believe it helps prevent hardening of arteries and the formation of kidney stones. This, however, still falls under the category of folklore.

But the fact remains that the healthful grapefruit is instrumental in helping one to lose weight. Now let's take a closer look at the other half of our formula: apple cider vinegar.

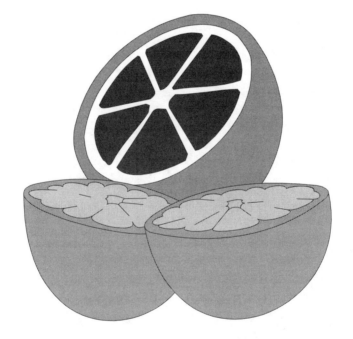

Chapter 3

Efficacious Apple Cider Vinegar

Before we explore the benefits of using apple cider vinegar as part of our weight loss diet, let's take a moment to acquaint ourselves with this marvelous substance.

Apple cider vinegar is one of several types of vinegar. Vinegar is derived from the French words vin (wine) and aigre (sour). It is a natural fermentation utilized even during biblical times that can be produced from various liquids that contain sugar. The one with which we are most familiar is white distilled vinegar. It's made from industrial alcohol. Another example in malt vinegar, yielded from malted barley, oats, corn or rye. Yet another example is wine vinegar, the end result of fermenting grapes. Apple cider vinegar, not surprisingly, is a vinegar created from the juice of apples.

The Health Benefits of Apples

The apple is an excellent ingredient for production into vinegar. A lot can be said about the nutritional value of this popular fruit. A medium apple including the peel (approximately two and three quarter inches in diameter) contains a multitude of substances essential for good health including 3 grams of fiber (particularly the kind known as pectin), 20 grams of carbohydrates, 160 milligrams of potassium, 10 milligrams of calcium, 8 milligrams of vitamin C, and 70 international units of vitamin A—within the confines of 80 calories. Yet it is virtually fat-free. It also contains little sodium.

Some Healthful Components of a Typical Apple

Serving size medium apple

- Fiber: 3 grams
- Carbohydrates: 20 grams
- Potassium: 160 milligrams
- Calcium: 10 milligrams
- Vitamin C: 8 milligrams
- Vitamin A: 70 International Units

Apples reduce the absorption of fat, thereby lowering blood cholesterol levels. At the same time, they raise good HDL cholesterol levels while diminishing concentrations of artery-clogging LDL. Apples are also capable of lowering blood pressure. In fact, according to a Yale University study, even the scent of apples is helpful in achieving lower blood pressure! Additionally, apples are good for the teeth, keep blood sugar levels steady, aid in maintaining regularity, and help in fighting colds. Generally speaking, those who consume more apples tend to be sick less.

The best part of all, thanks to its content of fiber, apples make one feel fuller than the equivalent dose of carbohydrate calories contained in other snack foods. In other words, apples can serve as an appetite suppressant!

How Apple Cider Vinegar is Made

Apple cider vinegar begins as ordinary cider after fresh, whole apples are pressed into juice. This sweet nutritious extract is allowed to age by being tightly sealed from the air. During this time the natural sugar that is present ferments to produce alcohol. Finally, the alcohol is exposed to the air and allowed to ferment again. On this second fermentation, the alcohol changes to acetic acid and water (apple cider vinegar). It's the acetic acid, by the way, that is responsible for apple cider vinegar's tart taste.

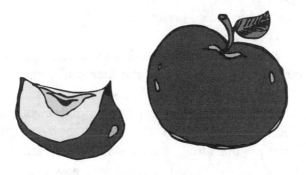

The fiber in apples helps one to feel full

Some Encouraging Words About Apple Cider Vinegar

Fortunately, apple cider vinegar still contains a large amount of the fundamental nutrients of the basic food from which it was produced; i. e., potassium, pectin, vitamins, minerals, and the like. Also present are other healthful substances, amino acids and enzymes, which are formed during the fermenting process. What's more, it possesses a long shelf life—and never requires refrigeration.

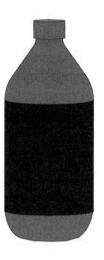

With good reason, apple cider vinegar enjoys an excellent reputation. We're learning to appreciate its properties just as those of ancient times did. It possesses a potent ability to disinfect, yet it's easy on the stomach. It's not only useful in destroying harmful bacteria inside the stomach and intestines, but aids the bladder and kidneys to function at peak efficiency. In other words, it helps the body clean itself of toxins. Among other things, apple cider vinegar also stimulates the immune system, and as stated earlier, keeps the metabolism in balance.

It has been said this golden liquid can remedy numerous afflictions such as asthma, hiccups, headaches, heartburn, and leg cramps. Some also believe that it is capable of clearing vision, improving hearing, and heightening one's mental processes. The most avid supporters even swear that it prolongs life! Some of these claims still fall under the category of folklore; many have now been medically proven.

> ### Learning From The Animals
>
> Animals know exactly how to administer treatment to themselves. Whenever they fall ill, they instinctively seek fermented fruit.

In any case, one fact is certain. Apple cider vinegar is a perfectly natural substance—and since it retains its ability to suppress the appetite just like the fruit from which it was produced, and because it regulates the metabolism, it is very useful for weight control.

How Apple Cider Vinegar Helps One to Lose Weight

Apple cider vinegar possesses the ability to help one embrace healthier eating habits. Not only does it suppress the appetite, a spoonful or two of apple cider vinegar taken regularly in a glass of water or other healthful liquid will also diminish your craving for certain edibles. You will find yourself losing the desire for sweets as well as for foods containing salt and fat.

In addition, this marvelous liquid improves cell respiration, which boosts the body's energy level. This process takes place in one of two ways. (1) The production of protein molecules within the cells is increased. This, in turn, leads to a rise in the metabolic rate, which is paramount for the control of weight. (2) The production of red blood cells is also increased, which means the absorption of iron from the digestive tract into the bloodstream is enhanced so it can be more expediently utilized. The bottom line: To create the energy required for this, fat must be burned—so it is extracted from the cells of the body's adipose tissue, i. e., a collection of fat cells, which are concentrated in the hips, stomach, and rear and upper thighs of an overweight person. In essence, you will find yourself losing weight just in the right spots. Furthermore, the fat that has been lost from these cells is not immediately replaced.

Rescue for Sugar-holics

Some have become so hooked on sugar that they can jokingly be called "sugar-holics". The prospect of giving up sweet foods for them seems hopeless. In their bid to beat the problem, many even resort to artificial sweeteners—unfortunate strategy since a question about their safety exists, and an irony because there is not that much saved in calories. They may skeptically ask, "How can apple cider vinegar curb my craving?"

The secret lies in the blood sugar level (glucose level) which frequently gets the blame for the development of a sugar addiction. When that level is low, one begins to feel irritated and nervous. If it gets low enough, fatigue or even depression will set in. It's at such times that one is seized by an urgent desire to devour fattening, sugar-laden snacks such as candy bars, cookies, cupcakes, and soda. Every time one begins to consume sweet foods such as these, the carbohydrates they contain are rapidly dispersed into the blood and transported to the brain and nerve cells. The blood sugar level rises, and he or she begins feeling better—but not without the cost of gaining too many of the wrong kind of calories. Furthermore, this "quick fix" will last only about 20 minutes, then the blood sugar level falls. Soon, a merciless cycle has begun.

Refined Sugar And Fat

The refined sugar in sweet snacks such as cookies, cakes, and candy bars that accompanies the large amount of fat usually contained in them does not contribute to weight gain in itself. However, it places stress on the adrenal glands, which are needed to help the thyroid regulate body weight.

Where does apple cider vinegar come in? It regulates the blood sugar level. Once that level is back in balance, one will no longer be plagued with this wild roller coaster ride of ups and downs. In addition, apple cider vinegar helps one acquire the taste for the natural foods such as fruits and vegetables that raise blood sugar levels more gradually—and, of course, which contain little fat.

Salt and Slimness: An Unlikely Mixture

Many are as crazy about salt as they are about sugar. French fries, sauces, meats, and the like always seem better when loaded with salt (the basic constituent of which is sodium). But we all know the truth. Salt and sliminess don't mix.

Don't get the wrong idea. Taking in a small amount of salt isn't going to hurt anyone. In fact, the body must have some sodium. In addition, salt supplies iodine (if iodized salt is used), another necessary component for a properly functioning body.

As outlined previously, however, sodium causes the body to retain more water by sucking it into the blood. The more salt consumed, the more water retained. Whenever an overabundance of salt is a part of the diet, weight can be gained in the stomach area because the sodium is absorbed into the nearby small intestine. Some carry almost 4½ pounds (2 kilograms) of excess weight because of this effect. Often this not only leaves one with more weight but with a bloated feeling as well.

Salt And Fatty Foods

The salt in fatty foods is often what is responsible for luring one toward those fatty foods. Fat itself has no taste.

Using apple cider vinegar as a salt substitute for as little as one week will help your taste buds adapt and halt your craving for salt. The characteristic flavors of nonfattening foods such as rice, beans, and potatoes will become more obvious to you. As a reinforcement and for variety's sake, you might also consider other alternatives to salt such as paprika, oregano leaves, and curry, not to mention pepper.

Apple Cider Vinegar And Salt

Apple cider vinegar is an attractive salt substitute. A spoonful in a bowl of homemade soup or as an ingredient in a homemade sauce will give you the impression that salt has been added.

Easy Does It

As you can see, apple cider vinegar is an excellent solution for weight control. Some may think, however, they can lose more weight faster by consuming larger quantities of it. The truth is, using more will not make you lose weight any faster because apple cider vinegar is designed for gradual steady reductions. And that's just as it should be. Losing too much weight too rapidly can be dangerous.

Those are the facts surrounding the magic of apple cider vinegar. Now let's get down to some serious business.

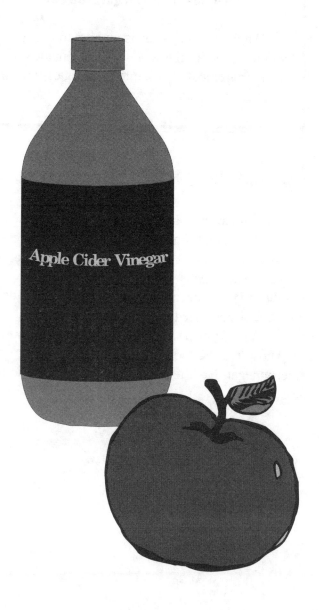

Part 2

The Game Plan

Chapter 4:

Delectable Drinks
To Soothe the Palate

Whenever the word "diet" comes up in conversation, one usually thinks more in terms of food than beverage. We know very well, though, that many colas, liquor, and the like are not your friends when it comes to losing weight. Although the fat content is not always a factor, they contribute little nourishment to the body. A typical 12 fluid ounce (360 grams) size cola, for instance, contains approximately 150 calories, yet little in the way of nutrients such as protein and vitamins that satisfy your hunger. Still, we usually find it difficult to give them up.

But don't despair. Besides the conventional low-fat beverages, there are a number of tasty nourishing drinks which can be whipped up from the kitchen that will fall right into your weight loss plan. They will add zest to any meal—and they include the use of none other than grapefruit and apple cider vinegar.

Before concerning ourselves with what we are going to chew on our diet, let's consider what we will be drinking. After all, drinks are in reality foods themselves.

Tips For Preparing Your Drinks

Before we proceed to the recipes, however, a few words about preparing your drinks are in order. Some can simply be mixed with a spoon. Those whose recipe calls for fresh whole fruits or vegetables, however, require one of several small appliances: a blender, a food processor or a juicer. A blender or processor purees (i. e., mashes) any produce put into it. You are left with a pulp which is a liquefied version of the original. This adds extra body to the drink that serves to help satisfy you. You receive the characteristic of a milk shake without the extra fat, and with nutritional benefits that a shake could never offer. A juicer, on the other hand, extracts most of the fiber from the juice. You are left with nothing more than a liquid. It still contains nourishment, but little in the way of substance. It suffices just fine as long as you include plenty of fiber in your meal by consuming lots of fresh fruits and vegetables.

When preparing recipes that call for any fresh fruit or vegetables, it is better not to substitute equivalents in juice form. While this can suit the purpose, the body derives much greater benefit out of the freshly-juiced food. And that brings up another point. While one is free to use purchased can or bottled juices in the recipes that do not specify whole produce, it is recommended that these juices also be obtained from the crushed whole fruit or vegetable.

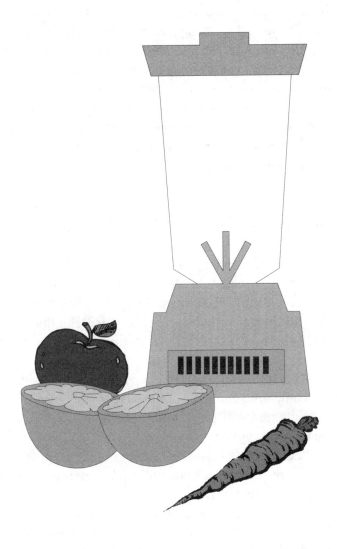

Drinks made with fresh fruits and vegetables are not only tasty and nourishing, they contain very little fat.

Drinks including these fresh fruits and vegetables should be consumed as soon as possible after preparation. The longer the delay, the more the nutritional value deteriorates. And the less nourishment you receive, the sooner your hunger pangs are going to return. If you absolutely must make a large quantity and won't be using the entire contents right away, at least store it in a dark airtight container in the refrigerator. This will help preserve the vitamin content. Even then, it is not advisable to keep it more than 24 hours.

Twelve Tasty Beverages Coming Up

Obviously we can pour ourselves a tall glass of grapefruit juice or include a teaspoon or two of apple cider vinegar in a tumbler of water. And certainly we can combine the vinegar with the grapefruit juice. But that would quickly become tiresome. Let's get imaginative—even exotic.

What follows are twelve recipes for producing drinks to accompany your meals. They all contain nutritious ingredients that will tickle your taste buds while helping you to lose weight.

Please note that all these recipes include apple cider vinegar, but sometimes you will find grapefruit juice absent. You will notice this particularly when vegetable juices appear among the ingredients. The reason is because it, like other fruits (with the exception of the apple), doesn't lend itself well to being mixed with vegetable juices. Therefore, to attain the maximum weight loss benefit from your diet, these beverages are more effective when used in conjunction with a meal in which grapefruit is a part. This is not to say that you will have to include both ingredients in every single case, but the more you do, the more advantage you will receive from the grapefruit and apple cider vinegar combination.

Now let's get down to business.

Cider Vinegar Fizz

Ingredients: carbonated water, 2 teaspoons of apple cider vinegar, 2 teaspoons of honey.

Instructions: Pour carbonated water into a glass. Stir in the apple cider vinegar and honey.

We start out with a variation to a simple theme. The carbonated water in this easily prepared beverage offers a little pep and is an excellent supplement for those having a difficult time giving up processed soft drinks. Meanwhile, the honey will help you forget about refined sugar. You will notice that the addition of an equal proportion of honey to apple cider vinegar causes it to resemble the taste of plain apple cider. In effect, you will be convinced you are drinking a carbonated apple cider beverage.

Remember that to get the full benefit of the apple cider vinegar, you should include it with a meal in which grapefruit is included.

Blueberry Mash

Ingredients: 2 cups of blueberry juice, 2 teaspoons of apple cider vinegar, 2 teaspoons of honey, 2 teaspoons of freshly-squeezed juice from a medium red grapefruit.

Instructions: Combine apple cider vinegar, honey, and grapefruit juice with blueberry juice and serve over crushed ice.

This makes a refreshingly different drink. The blueberry is another excellent fruit useful for weight control, thanks to its healthy content of potassium and small contribution of sodium. It also contributes a lot of pectin to the cause. Therefore, the best scenario is make your juice from fresh blueberries using a blender or food processor. That way you will retain the full quantity of fiber.

In addition, it might be worthwhile to note that Swedish researchers have discovered blueberries are loaded with chemicals known as anthocyanosides, which kill *E. coli* bacteria!

Strawberry Nectar

Ingredients: 2 cups of strawberry juice, 3 teaspoons of red grapefruit juice, 2 teaspoons of apple cider vinegar, 2 teaspoons of honey, nutmeg.

Instructions: Mix strawberry juice with grapefruit juice, apple cider vinegar, and honey. Add a dash of nutmeg.

This is an easy-to-make beverage with a somewhat exotic flavor. Like the blueberry, strawberries are strong on potassium and possess a healthy amount of fiber, mostly in the form of pectin. Strawberries are also rich in vitamin A and C, and contain many minerals. It's certainly a pleasant bonus to combine with the beneficial effects of grapefruit and apple cider vinegar.

What a great idea for a breakfast drink.

Tropic Delight on the Grapefruit Rocks

Ingredients: 8 ounces (225 grams) of fresh fruit of your choice, ¼ liter of pineapple juice, 1 teaspoon of apple cider vinegar, 1 teaspoon of honey, red grapefruit juice.

Instructions: Squeeze enough grapefruit juice to freeze into ice. Wash and dice the 8 ounces of fruit, then process into juice. Blend juice with other ingredients. Serve over grapefruit ice.

This drink is fun because you can vary its flavor by including any fruit you like. The pineapple juice it contains is especially beneficial because of the all-important enzyme bromelain, which speeds up the digestion of protein-rich foods, by efficiently metabolizing (breaking down) their amino acids. This drink is an especially good choice after eating any dish which includes animal products. For best results in this case, the drink should be consumed a half hour after the meal. Keep in mind, however, that taking in a lot of animal products is not a good idea for those attempting to lose weight.

Pineapple is also noted for its content of manganese, a vital part of certain enzymes needed to metabolize carbohydrates as well as protein. In addition, the vitamin C and bioflavonoids in the pineapple work just like those in the grapefruit. Take a few sips, then close your eyes and imagine a beautiful Hawaiian setting.

Vinegar Punch

Ingredients: ¼ *liter of cherry juice,* ¼ *liter of grapefruit juice, 16 ounces (450 grams) of fresh raspberries, 1 liter of carbonated water, 2 teaspoons of honey, 2 tablespoons of apple cider vinegar.*

Instructions: Juice raspberries and pour into pitcher. Add cherry and grapefruit juices, carbonated water, honey, and apple cider vinegar. Stir and serve.

These fruits make a lively blend and are loaded with vitamin C and bioflavonoids, as is, of course, the apple cider vinegar. Vitamin A comes into play again here with the cherry juice. The cherry juice also contains potassium and darker cherries are richer in potassium than the lighter variety. If you choose to puree or juice fresh cherries, purchase the sweet variety. The sour kind are more disposed for canning. This recipe not only makes a tasty treat any time, but is an excellent choice for a party drink as well. And it just might become addictive.

Vinegar Vegetable Cocktail

Ingredients: 1 can of low-sodium vegetable juice, 1 teaspoon of barley powder, 1 tablespoon of apple cider vinegar.

Instructions: Pour apple cider vinegar and barley powder into juice. Stir and serve.

The apple cider vinegar in this simple, but effective recipe is efficient at activating the nutrients of the vegetable juice, thereby making it possible for the body to utilize them to their utmost. The barley powder provides extra life-giving chlorophyll, which produces a natural cleansing effect within the body that helps free clogged arteries.

You may prefer to make your own vegetable juice to use for this drink, since it will be much fresher than a canned product.

Vinegar Tomato Cocktail

Ingredients: 4 tomatoes, ½ stalk celery, 1 tablespoon of apple cider vinegar.

Instructions: Wash, core and dice the tomatoes. Wash and slice celery. Combine in blender and process. Then add apple cider vinegar to juice. Stir and serve.

This, of course, is a superb choice for tomato juice aficionados. You will get a beverage rich in potassium that will give you over one third of your daily requirement of vitamins A and C. Again, remember, to maximize weight loss results, this is a drink that should be used in conjunction with meals which include grapefruit.

Citrus Tea

Ingredients: 1 quart (approximately 1 liter) of camomile tea, 1 tablespoon of lemon juice, 1 teaspoon of grapefruit juice, 3 tablespoons of honey, 1 tablespoon of apple cider vinegar, 1 basil leaf.

Instructions: Mix tea with lemon juice, grapefruit juice, honey, and apple cider vinegar. Add basil leaf.

This is a great selection for tea lovers. The ascorbic acid and citric acid contained in the lemon and grapefruit juice goes well with the acetic acid of the vinegar to encourage the production of gastric acid which, in turn, bolsters the utilization of protein. Meanwhile, the herbal tea cleans out the intestines and lessens the absorption of fat into the blood.

Vinegar Fruit Soda

Ingredients: 2 cups water, ½ cup dried apricots, 1 cup grape juice, 1 cup apple juice, 3 teaspoons honey, 3 teaspoons apple cider vinegar, 2 teaspoons of freshly-squeezed juice from a medium red grapefruit.

Instructions: Pour water in pan. Add dried apricots. Bring to boil. Add grape, apple, and grapefruit juice plus honey along with apple cider vinegar. Heat again while stirring, then serve.

The apricots provide a special treat and makes this drink unique. Apricots are a rich source of vitamin A, rivaled only by the cantaloupe. They also contain iron as well as potassium, which can not only draw excess water from the body, but provides energy and stamina.

The grape juice, as well as the apple juice, is a good source of chromium. This trace mineral promotes the burning of unnecessary fat. In addition, it is essential for keeping blood sugar stable, which as stated earlier, halts the craving for the wrong kind of foods. (It is a bitter irony that the excess consumption of unhealthful sweets prevents the absorption of chromium, which makes the matter of blood sugar instability all the worse.)

A delicious, tangy treat, this warm beverage is excellent for those miserably cold winter days. It is also a great idea for holiday occasions. Now pour yourself a glass and curl up by the fire.

Spicy Carrot Blend

Ingredients: 12 ounces (360 grams) carrot juice, ½ teaspoon celery salt, ½ teaspoon pepper, 1 tablespoon apple cider vinegar.

Instructions: Mix carrot juice with apple cider vinegar. Add a dash of celery salt and pepper. (It is recommended that you use a juicer for this recipe if using whole carrots. Hard vegetables such as carrots will not process properly without adding extra liquid.)

This could just as easily be called the vitamin A drink. In fact, its beta carotene content far exceeds the recommended daily requirement. It's also a good source of vitamin C, vitamin E, potassium, iron, calcium, and phosphorus. What's more, the carrot juice is easy to digest. This is an excellent beverage for consumption any time, but for optimum figure-trimming results should be consumed along with a meal containing grapefruit.

Cucumber Carrot Cocktail

Ingredients: ½ *cucumber, 4 carrots, 1 tea-spoon of parsley, 1 tablespoon dill, 1 tablespoon apple cider vinegar, a dash of celery salt.*

Instructions: *Peel and dice cucumber half. Dice carrots. Place in juicer. Add parsley, dill, apple cider vinegar and celery salt. Mix and serve. (It is recommended that you use a juicer for this recipe. Hard vegetables such as carrots will not process properly without adding extra liquid.)*

The substances contained in the parsley and dill in this beverage work together with the apple cider vinegar to clean out the small intestine and colon of unwanted bacteria and fungi. This stimulates intestinal peristalsis (wavelike movement of the intestinal walls) which results in a swifter excretion of food particles. This, in turn, means less fat can be absorbed in the intestines.

Tangy Banana Pick-Me-Up

Ingredients: 1 orange, ½ red grapefruit, 1 banana, 2 teaspoons apple cider vinegar, 2 teaspoons honey.

Instructions: Peel the orange, grapefruit, and banana. Separate sections of citrus fruits and chop banana. Place together in a blender along with apple cider vinegar and honey. If you desire a colder drink, freeze the banana first. (Do not use a juicer. Due to their softness, bananas are extremely difficult, if not impossible to juice.)

This thick, creamy beverage, reminiscent of a milk shake, is especially rich in potassium, as well as other minerals because of the banana. In fact, in regard to mineral content, the banana is second only to strawberries. The banana also contains the amino acid tryptophan. Needless to say, this drink also offers a generous supply of vitamin C. Because of its rich texture, it is especially efficient at giving one a feeling of fullness. It's not bad for the privilege of experiencing the characteristic of a milk shake, without the burden of extra fat calories.

By now you have probably caught on that you don't have to adhere strictly to the above recipes. They can be altered in numerous ways. In fact, there are many other combinations that can be utilized to make excellent beverages in which grapefruit juice and/or apple cider vinegar can be included. You might prefer to blend strawberry and banana or carrot and apple. Feel free to put your ingenuity to work. With a little creativity, you can invent numerous other drinks that will be both satisfying and nutritious— and virtually fat-free!

Now let's consider what we will be putting into our plate.

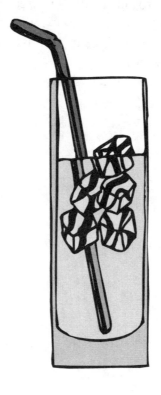

Chapter 5:

The Express Diet

For those who do not need to lose much weight, or for those who are short on patience, or who envision a lengthier diet as dismal, this three-day plan will likely be made to order.

There will be little to displease vegetarians. As with any worthwhile diet, it will go heavy on vegetables, fruits, and grains, and light on animal products, which contribute far too much fat. Processed sweet snacks on the order of cookies, pies, candy and the like will not be included because they all too often contain animal products, refined sugar, and flour. There will be no alcohol or caffeine, as alcohol can deplete the body of potassium and other important chemicals, while caffeine can deplete nutrients such as thiamine (vitamin B_1), vitamin C, calcium, and chromium as well as potassium. Of course, our diet will include an appropriate share of grapefruit and apple cider vinegar.

The Facts About Fat

Although fat is considered a bitter enemy of the overweight, it is actually essential to the body. It provides energy, functions as a barrier to keep out harmful microbes, transports vitamins throughout the body, helps build cell walls and much more. In fact, the brain is actually composed of 60% fat. But you don't need much, and you can get all you require in the modest amount supplied in fruits, vegetables, and whole grains.

In addition, the fats found in these foods are the right kind for the body. They consist mostly of the unsaturated variety. These healthy fats, known as essential fats, are largely absent from animal products, which chiefly contain saturated fats. Interestingly, unsaturated fats can help stop craving for fatty foods that are not healthy.

The following are suggestions for what to eat and drink for all three meals of the Express Diet and any snacks you might desire:

Breakfast:

Citrus-Melon Eye-Opener

Ingredients: 1 white grapefruit, ½ canteloupe, 1 slice of whole wheat bread.

Instructions: Peel grapefruit, separate sections and enjoy along with canteloupe and bread. Toast bread if desired.

Suggested Beverage:
Vinegar Tomato Cocktail

This is a simple meal that contains little in the way of fat calories. But you will be getting a lot of potassium and a generous amount of vitamin A, not to mention all the vitamin C your body will require for the day. The bread will provide your serving of grain, with whole wheat or any whole grain being a better choice than the white variety, which has had bleaching agents used during its manufacture.

Fruit Salad Delight

Ingredients: 1 apple, 1 banana, 1 grapefruit, 1 cup of low- or no-fat yogurt, 1 tablespoon of almond slivers.

Instructions: Chop apple. Peel and chop banana. Place in serving dish. Then peel and separate grapefruit sections and add to the other fruit. Cut into finer pieces if desired. Mix with the yogurt and sprinkle almonds on top.

Suggested Beverage:
Vinegar Vegetable Cocktail

We have already become well acquainted with the apple, banana, and grapefruit. You'll certainly take in no significant fat calories with this trio no matter how much you eat. The only thing we afford ourselves in this meal in the way of an animal product is the yogurt—and the low-fat version will not contribute significantly to the fat content of the dish. The almonds, do contain a certain amount of fat, but most of the fat they do contain exists in the form of the unsaturated variety, not the saturated kind chiefly found in considerable quantities in animal products. They are also a source of calcium. And as does any nut, almonds provide needed protein—at that, in the most natural way because they are not an animal product but originate from the same source as the fruits—a tree.

Egg—Wheat Combo

Ingredients: 1 egg, 1 slice of whole wheat bread, 2 romaine lettuce leaves, 3 small red radishes, salt, paprika.

Instructions: Hard boil the egg, then peel and slice. Chop radishes into quarters. Add lettuce, season to taste with salt and paprika. Serve on dish. Toast bread if desired.

Suggested Beverage:
Strawberry Nectar

This meal is designed for those who are accustomed to an egg breakfast. The egg is the only thing that will contribute any significant amount of fat. The radishes contain a generous amount of potassium and a small quantity of Vitamin C. What otherwise might be considered a light breakfast, will be enhanced by the strawberry drink. It will prove more filling if you use the fresh whole fruit which has been mashed in a blender or processor.

Lunch:

Salad—Potato Special

Ingredients: 2 leaves of crisp fresh lettuce, 2 stalks of celery, 1 slice of white onion, 1 carrot, ½ dozen cherry tomatoes, 1 red bell pepper, 1 tablespoon of olive oil, 1 teaspoon of apple cider vinegar, 1 teaspoon of lemon juice, 1 large potato, butter.

Instructions: Slice lettuce, celery, onion, carrot, and bell pepper. Add tomatoes. Make a salad dressing by mixing olive oil, apple cider vinegar and lemon juice, then apply to vegetables. Bake the potato. Add butter.

Suggested Beverage:
Citrus Tea

This is a delightfully tasty meal with plenty of nourishment. The only drawback for weight watchers here besides butter is the olive oil. But olive oil possesses a redeeming value in that it contains a lot of the essential fatty acids alpha-linolenic (omega-3) as well as linoleic (omega-6), and has been found to lower cholesterol levels—and blood pressure. Butter is a better choice than margarine because margarine contains more saturated fat.

Colorful Vegetable Plate

Ingredients: 1 serving of shredded carrots, 1 teaspoon of raisins, 1 serving of pineapple chunks, 1 serving of green beans, 1 tomato, 1 ear of corn, pepper.

Instructions: Prepare a carrot salad using shredded carrots, raisins, and pineapple chunks. Slice tomato. Shuck and wash corn. Serve salad with green beans, tomato and corn. Pepper to taste.

Suggested Beverage:
Tangy Banana Pick-Me-Up

There's nothing fattening about this meal. Yet its colorful and palatable. It is not necessary to cook the corn. A good ear of this grain will be tender and tasty as is. It contains a lot of potassium, but is not high in sodium, and is a respectable source of iron as well as zinc. Green beans contain the fiber lignin, which helps speed food through the stomach. They also contain cellulose, another fiber that moves waste through the colon more rapidly, thereby assisting in the prevention of constipation.

For a more nutritional salad, shred fresh whole carrots rather than using the pre-shredded kind.

Salmon—Celery Supreme

Ingredients: *4 ounces of canned salmon, 2 celery stalks, 1 green bell pepper, 1 roma tomato, 1 thin slice of purple onion, lemon slice.*

Instructions: *Chop bell pepper. Slice tomato. Dice onion. Mix onion with salmon. Garnish with lemon slice. Serve with celery, bell pepper, and tomato.*

Suggest Beverage:
Vinegar Punch

The salmon contains fat, but this fat comes in the form of essential fatty acids, particularly omega-3. It is very tasty—especially when onion is added. Celery provides a good source of fiber and gives you the sodium your body requires without over-doing it. As for bell pepper, it actually rivals orange juice for its content of vitamin C.

Dinner:

Raw Veggie Platter

Ingredients: broccoli, cauliflower, radishes, cucumbers, carrots, red cabbage, a low-fat or fat-free bottled salad dressing containing cider vinegar, 1 slice whole wheat bread.

Instructions: Chop broccoli, cauliflower, radishes, cucumbers, carrots, and cabbage in the amount desired. Pour on salad dressing. Serve with bread. Toast bread if desired.

Suggested Beverage:
Vinegar Fruit Soda

This is a delightful meal for those who like (or are in a mood for) a crunchy dish. And in its uncooked state, all the nutrition these fine foods offer is retained. Fiber plays a big role. Not only does the cabbage provide its share of fiber (even somewhat more so than the white variety), it gives you a large portion of the recommended daily allowance of vitamin C. Combined with the other vegetables and the fruit drink, you should receive more than the full daily dosage of this important vitamin.

Fruit in the Cottage

Ingredients: 1 banana, ½ grapefruit, 1 pear, 1 serving of cottage cheese, 1 teaspoon of honey, 1 teaspoon of chopped dates, 2 slices of whole wheat bread.

Instructions: Dice banana, grapefruit, and pear. Mix honey in cottage cheese. Mix fruit in cottage cheese. Top with chopped dates. Serve with bread. Toast bread if desired.

Suggested Beverage:
Cucumber Carrot Cocktail

For fruit lovers, this light meal will prove especially enjoyable. As with any dried fruit, the dates add an extra zing of sweetness. Dates include potassium and a substantial amount of dietary fiber. And not unlike the apple, the pear's content of fiber in the form of pectin is top-notch. Meanwhile, the cucumber carrot drink will supply you with lots of vegetable nourishment.

Tasty Tofu Plate

Ingredients: 2 slices of firm tofu, 1 egg, 4 large lettuce leafs, 1 medium tomato, 1 slice of whole wheat bread, 1 teaspoon of wheat germ, 1 teaspoon of apple cider vinegar, 2 teaspoons of olive oil, butter.

Instructions: Boil egg and slice. Chop lettuce and tomato and place in a bowl. Mix apple cider vinegar and olive oil, then combine with tomato and lettuce. Finally, place egg slices on top. Butter bread, sprinkle on wheat germ, and serve with tofu and salad.

Suggested Beverage:
Tropic Delight on the Grapefruit Rocks

Tofu, derived from soy beans, is an excellent substitute for meat. Although bland, it has the tendency to take on the flavor of whatever food (and spices) is prepared with it. That makes it very versatile. (There are also flavored varieties from which to choose.) It can even be mixed with other ingredients to make a salad dressing. Although it contains fat, little of that fat is saturated and it provides a lot of iron, calcium, and protein.

The wheat germ will give you a more complete grain, since the highly perishable germ of the grain used to make bread is normally removed, even in products that imply on the label that the whole grain was used with terms such as "whole wheat", "rye", or "seven-grain".

> **Snacks:**
>
> • Any fresh fruit, such as apples and grapefruits
> • Any dried fruit, such as raisins
> • A raw carrot
> • Dill pickles
> • Additional servings of any of the suggested drinks

Express Diet Summary

You have undoubtedly noticed by now just how scarce the animal products are in the above menu suggestions. Of course, you know the reason. With a weight loss plan of such short duration, one should lean as heavily toward low-fat foods as possible in order to achieve meaningful results.

If you do not feel such meals are enough for you, have another helping, particularly of any of the fruits and vegetables. In fact, feel free to splurge on these. They will add no significant fat calories no matter how many you eat. Hint: Fruit is always a good standby for those who feel slighted without dessert.

Also, don't overlook water during your diet. You should drink plenty of it. Eight 8 ounce glasses is recommended. Water is essential for transporting nutrients to its cells and for carrying away toxins and wastes. You won't have to fear retaining an excessive amount of it when your level of sodium and potassium is in balance. As renown physician Earl Mindell expresses it, "Water fills you up without filling you out".

For those who do not prefer the design of this diet plan, you can afford yourself a few extra amenities and take a little longer to see your result as you will see in the following chapter.

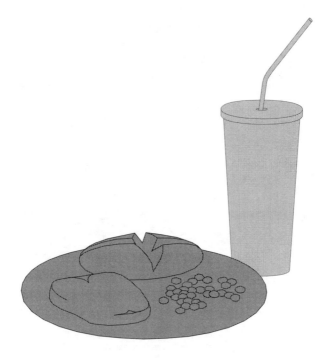

Chapter 6:

The Intermediate Diet

For those who want to spread out their game plan somewhat, this diet plan will probably work better. It will extend over a ten-day period. You will still see plenty of fruits, vegetables, and whole grains, but a few more animal products will also be allowed. Emphasis, however, will still be on the former. No foodstuffs made with refined sugar and animal products will be included, nor will alcohol or anything containing caffeine. Of course, you will still receive your share of grapefruit and apple cider vinegar.

Protein: How Much is Enough?

There's no question about it, protein is essential to the body. Among other things, it builds muscle, which is necessary in helping you to burn calories. A lack of protein can create brain chemistry imbalances. This tends to induce feelings such as depression and anxiety, which can in turn lead to "emotional" eating habits.

However, some still hold onto the mistaken belief that eliminating meat and other animal products from one's diet will deprive his or her body of its required amount of protein. Not so. A balanced supply of fruits, vegetables, whole grains, and beans will provide all the protein needed.

On the other hand, too much protein presents a problem of its own. Excess protein increases the excretion of calcium. This, in turn, can lead to osteoporosis. The only way one can overdose on protein, however, is to get it through the high content present in animal products. Not only will healthy foods such as vegetables give you *all* the protein needed, it will not give you *more* than you need.

The following are suggestions for what to eat and drink for all three meals while participating in the intermediate diet, as well as any snacks you might desire:

Breakfast:

Fruit and Cereal Special

Ingredients: A low-fat whole-grain cereal, skim milk, 1 grapefruit, 1 banana.

Instructions: Pour cereal into bowl. Add milk. Chop banana and add. Peel grapefruit and eat on the side.

Suggested Beverage:
Spicy Carrot Blend

Cereal, of course, is produced from a grain. It will not only help you to get the required grain the body needs, but when supplemented with fruit such as a banana, you will be receiving some excellent nutrition. As we have already established, bananas are strong in the potassium department. Your fat calories from the milk will obviously be reduced by using the low-fat variety. Meanwhile, the carrot drink will give you a significant amount of vitamins.

Poached Egg Dish with Carrot

Ingredients: 1 egg, 1 slice of whole grained bread, butter, salt, pepper, 1 carrot, a dash of apple cider vinegar, a dash of olive oil.

Instructions: Poach egg. Salt and pepper to taste. Toast bread, add butter. Scrape carrot, then dress with apple cider vinegar and olive oil. Serve and enjoy.

Suggested Beverage:
A tall glass of grapefruit juice

This is an egg breakfast with a twist—a spiced up carrot. That makes it a meal good in vitamin content and it fits in nicely with those who find it difficult to do without their morning egg. In might be added, that although a large poached egg contains roughly 5 grams of fat, it also provides protein. Unless you consume a large number of eggs or suffer from coronary artery disease, they should not pose a big problem.

Tart Fruit Salad

Ingredients: 1 grapefruit, 1 kiwi, 1 apple.

Instructions: Peel grapefruit, separate sections, and slice. Peel kiwi and slice. Slice apple. Combine ingredients and enjoy.

Suggested Beverage:
Vinegar Tomato Cocktail

Nothing really fancy here, but there's plenty of nourishment. The Kiwi, whose flavor seems somewhat cross between a strawberry and a pineapple, contributes lots of vitamin C as do the other two fruits. It's a great choice for those who like to begin their day with fruit. The tart flavor will really wake up the taste buds, too. It will also supply energy—the natural way—and the more energy one has, the more active he or she has a tendency to be—and the more fat will be burned.

Lunch:

Cheese Special Plus

Ingredients: 1 slice of low- or no-fat cheese, 2 slices of whole wheat bread, 1 slice of fresh tomato, 1 romaine lettuce leaf, 2 white radishes, 1 green bell pepper, ½ red grapefruit.

Instructions: Slice bell pepper. Place cheese between bread slices with tomato and lettuce. Enjoy along with radishes and bell pepper on the side. Serve grapefruit half for dessert.

Suggested Beverage:
Cider Vinegar Fizz

The combination of tomato and cheese makes a tasty sandwich. The generous moisture in the tomato will help make up for the absence of fattening condiments. Radishes give the meal an extra bite. In addition to calcium, chromium is found in cheese, which as mentioned earlier, is essential for keeping blood sugar stable. The downside on cheese, however, is that many low-fat varieties also contain phosphate, which is thought to interfere with the body's absorption of calcium. Fat will not even be a factor with it, though, unless you haven't chosen a no-fat product.

Also, please note that romaine is a better choice than the popular iceberg lettuce. The iceberg variety degrades more slowly and may contribute to constipation. Any of the other green leaf as well as red leaf lettuce are also better choices.

Turkey Sandwich with Homemade "Potato Chips"

Ingredients: 2 slices of white meat turkey without skin, 2 slices rye bread, 2 whole dill pickles, 1 medium raw new potato, 1 teaspoon fat reduced mayonnaise, garlic salt, paprika.

Instructions: Apply mayonnaise to bread and add turkey. Cut unpeeled potato in thin slices. Sprinkle with garlic salt, and paprika. Serve sandwich with pickles and these homemade "potato chips".

Suggested Beverage:
Citrus Tea

As far as meat is concerned, turkey is an excellent lower-fat alternative. It contains less fat than red meats and white turkey meat is less fattening than dark turkey meat. The raw sliced potatoes offer a crispiness just like conventional potato chips, yet with a pleasing amount of moisture. The garlic salt, and paprika will dress up the flavor. And unlike processed potato chips, these fresh slices retain all the original nutrients—including potassium, protein, vitamin B complex, calcium, and iron—and, of course, no consideration as to fat.

Veggie Plate Plus

Ingredients: 1 serving of shredded cabbage, 1 teaspoon of currants, 1 serving of English peas, 1 tomato, 1 ear of corn, 1 teaspoon fat reduced mayonnaise, 1 slice of pumpernickel bread, 1 pat of butter, salt, pepper, 1 serving of apple sauce.

Instructions: Mix mayonnaise into cabbage and add currants to make slaw. Slice tomato. Shuck and wash corn. Place slaw in plate with English peas, tomato slices, and corn. Salt and pepper lightly. Serve with buttered bread, then have apple sauce for dessert.

Suggested Beverage:
Vinegar Punch

This is another colorful and palatable dish. The only fat you will be getting will come from the mayonnaise and butter. You will get your share of potassium from the corn, as well as iron and zinc. The peas are something else to be praised. They possess virtually no sodium, cholesterol or fat, but a generous amount of soluble fiber along with vitamins A and C. For a more nutritional salad, shred fresh whole cabbage rather than using the pre-shredded kind.

Dinner:

Rice and Bean Combo

Ingredients: 1 serving of brown rice, 1 serving of pinto beans, 1 serving of sodium-free vegetable soup, 1 slice of whole wheat bread, 1 banana, 1 teaspoon of apple cider vinegar, pepper.

Instructions: Cook rice and beans. Pour soup into bowl, heat and stir in apple cider vinegar. Sprinkled pepper on beans and rice. Serve with soup and bread. Serve banana for dessert—or freeze it peeled and serve as a low-fat popsicle.

Suggested Beverage:
Blueberry Mash

This is a high protein dish—without the fat. The beans provide most of that protein. In fact, a full cup of beans of any kind contain more protein than can be derived from a fast-food hamburger. Beans are also loaded with complex carbohydrates, potassium, iron, and thiamine (vitamin B_1) as well as fiber. In regard to quantity of fiber, pintos top the list of all varieties of beans. And don't take the pepper for granted. It contains a noteworthy amount of chromium.

Adding apple cider vinegar to the soup will lend to it a salty flavor, satisfying any craving for salt or salt-laced foods. Homemade soup, of course, is the best choice for optimum nutritional value.

Spaghetti with Tofu

Ingredients: 1 serving of whole grain spaghetti, 1 tomato, 1 garlic glove, ½ teaspoon of oregano leaves, 1 generous slice of tofu, 1 bell pepper, 1 celery stalk, 1 carrot, 1 teaspoon of canola oil, 1 teaspoon of apple cider vinegar.

Instructions: Prepare spaghetti dish, cooking in tomato, garlic, and oregano leaves. Remove from heat. Chop tofu slice into small pieces and mix in with spaghetti. Finely chop bell pepper, celery and carrot. Mix canola oil and apple cider vinegar and pour onto vegetables as a dressing. Serve with spaghetti dish.

Suggested Beverage:
Tropic Delight on the Grapefruit Rocks

Spaghetti, as with any pasta, is chocked full of minerals. This includes manganese, iron, copper, phosphorus, magnesium, and zinc. In fact, 2 cups of pasta according to the American Institute of Baking, provides 31% of the Recommended Dietary Allowance of manganese. Interestingly, tests have shown that it retains these minerals well during cooking. Meanwhile, fat and sodium stand at a minimum.

Garlic contains a noteworthy amount of potassium. It helps reduce cholesterol, triglycerides, and blood pressure. The canola oil contains fat, but it comes primarily in the form of omega-3 and omega-6. Omega-6, among other things, helps prevent adverse effects on the adrenal and the thyroid glands.

Chicken Salad—Vegetable Platter

Ingredients: 1 cup of chicken salad, 1 serving of cooked sweet potatoes, 1 serving of cooked broccoli, 1 slice rye bread, pepper.

Instructions: Serve chicken salad, sweet potatoes, and broccoli with rye bread.

Suggested Beverage:
Vinegar Fruit Soda

When considering meat, chicken is another lower-fat alternative similar to turkey. Although you will receive some fat, you will also be getting protein. The sweet potato, just as the carrot, offers a large dose of beta carotene containing vitamin A. Its also a liberal contributor of vitamin C, fiber, and potassium. A lot of potassium and vitamin C is also supplied by the broccoli.

> **Snacks:**
>
> • Any fresh fruit, such as apples, grapefruits, and oranges
> • Any dried fruit, such as raisins and dates
> • A raw carrot
> • Dill pickles
> • A slice of whole grain bread
> • A small serving of unsalted nuts
> • Additional servings of any of the suggested drinks

Intermediate Diet Summary

You undoubtedly detected an increase in the variety of meats in this diet. However, they are lean meats, more suited for a weight-loss diet. In a ten-day period, they should not add significantly to your overall fat content if they are used reasonably. Turkey and chicken, along with fish should satisfy those who don't want to be left without meat. Most of your diet will still consist of fruits and vegetables, both on the plate and in the glass.

If this plan is still too drastic for you, however, and you would like to really take your time losing weight, read on.

Chapter 7

The Extended Diet

For those who desire a longer-range plan for their diet, this is it. The Extended Diet will stretch over a 30-day period. Although confined to a reasonable level, we'll take a few more liberties with animal products. There will be more occasion to butter our bread and adorn our meals with cheese. We'll afford ourselves a little more increase of meat. The only things for which there will be no room are products containing refined sugar, as well as any alcohol or caffeine. Fruits and vegetables, of course, will still be prevalent along with grapefruit and apple cider vinegar.

Calorie Quality

Most have been fooled by conventional diets (those that focus solely on the reduction of caloric intake). Estimates are that 95% of them end in failure. Why?

The success formula for losing weight clearly does not rest with the number of calories consumed. The caloric count is not a measure of how fattening a food is. Some foods possess fewer calories composed of fat. Other contain a higher portion of fat calories. For instance, the percentage of calories from fat of chuck roast is 51%. The ratio for potatoes is less than 1%! You would, therefore, have to consume a frightfully large volume of potatoes as compared to that of the meat to take in the same number of fat calories.

Obviously, then, when two different foods contain the same amount of calories, this does not necessarily mean they are equally as fattening. One might say, it's the quality of calories that counts.

The following are suggestions for what to eat and drink for all three meals while participating in the Extended Diet, as well as any snacks you might desire:

Breakfast:

Sweet-N-Sour Fruit Salad

Ingredients: 1 grapefruit half, 1 orange, 1 apple, 1 teaspoon raisins, 2 teaspoons chopped pecans, 1 cup of low- or no-fat yogurt.

Instructions: Chop apple and place in serving dish. Then peel and separate grapefruit and orange sections. Cut into finer pieces if desired. Then add to apple. Mix with the yogurt and sprinkle raisins and pecans on top.

Suggested Beverage:
Cucumber Carrot Cocktail

This is just suited for those who like their fruit in the morning. Of course, our old standby the grapefruit is included. The citrus fruit along with the raisins give the dish a lively sweet and sour effect. The yogurt will not be a big factor if you at least stick to the low-fat variety. No-fat, of course, will be of greater help. Pecans possess slightly more fat than the almonds suggested in the Express Diet, but not a whole lot more—and they are a good source of thiamine (Vitamin B_1), which plays its part to help stabilize blood sugar.

Egg and More

Ingredients: 1 egg, 1 tomato, 1 slice of low-fat cheese, 1 serving of black beans, 1 serving of spinach leaves, 1 celery stalk, 1 slice whole wheat bread.

Instructions: Boil egg, then peel and slice. Slice tomato and serve along with egg, cheese, spinach, celery and beans. Toast bread and serve with dish.

Suggested Beverage:
Strawberry Nectar

In this dish we have the pleasure of an egg and cheese. The cheese will not be a big factor if it is low-fat. Meanwhile, the fresh vegetables contribute lots of nutrition. The tomato, in itself, (botanically speaking, a fruit rather than a vegetable) provides a vitamin C content which is 50% of the recommended daily allowance. It also contains potassium and its share of fiber. Tomatoes are also an excellent source of vitamin A—not from beta carotene, but another carotene known as lycopene. Spinach, as well as other dark green leafy vegetables such as kale, chard, collard, mustard greens and dandelion contain omega-3, which helps raise the metabolic rate so that calories can be burned at a more brisk pace. It also assists the kidneys in eliminating excess water from the tissues. And as for the beans, they provide plenty of protein. Who says you can't eat beans for breakfast?

Strawberry—Banana Cereal

Ingredients: 1 cup of low-fat cereal, low-fat milk, 1 banana, 6 medium strawberries, ½ grapefruit.

Instructions: Pour cereal into bowl and add milk. Chop banana and add to cereal along with strawberries. Eat grapefruit on the side.

Suggested Beverage:
Vinegar Vegetable Cocktail

For cereal lovers, this is a good selection. The cereal helps to furnish your body's requirement for grain and the healthful fruits do their thing to nourish with precious little in the way of fat content.

Lunch:

Soup and Sandwich Combo

Ingredients: 1 can of low-sodium vegetable soup, 1 thin slice of lean roast beef, 1 teaspoon of mustard, 2 slices of whole grain bread, 1 tomato slice, 1 lettuce leaf, 1 teaspoon of apple cider vinegar.

Instructions: Pour soup into bowl. Stir in apple cider vinegar. Apply mustard to bread and add roast beef, tomato, and lettuce.

Suggested Beverage:
Tropic Delight on the Grapefruit Rocks

There's nothing that goes together like soup and sandwich. Here, we are even affording ourselves some roast beef. We'll get our vegetables largely this time from what's in the soup. Homemade soup, of course, is best. The touch of apple cider vinegar in the soup serves as a excellent salt substitute. Since many canned soups contain sodium, that's all the more reason the make your soup right from the kitchen. Also, using mustard that contains cider vinegar is the best choice.

Tuna Treat

Ingredients: 1 can of tuna fish, 1 stalk of celery, 1 small cucumber, 6 olives, 1 lemon wedge, 1 teaspoon of fat reduced mayonnaise, ½ teaspoon of apple cider vinegar, ½ teaspoon of vegetable oil, 1 slice of rye bread, 1 pat of butter.

Instructions: Place tuna in a plate. Chop celery and add to tuna, then mix in mayonnaise. Add lemon wedge. Slice cucumber and dress with apple cider vinegar and vegetable oil. Toast bread and butter it. Serve with tuna, cucumber slices, and olives.

Suggested Beverage:
A tall glass of grapefruit juice

The tuna is tasty and the celery gives it a nice texture while supplying a lot of fiber. The cucumber furnishes a large amount of potassium as well as manganese and sulfur. The olives, although they contain some fat, are immensely nourishing—and most of the fat they do contain is unsaturated. To minimize the fat content of this meal, use tuna that has been packed in water—not oil. Also consider substituting a lemon vinaigrette for the mayo. Most vegetable oils will do for a dressing, but the best seem to be canola and olive oil.

King Size Salad

Ingredients: 1 bell pepper, 1 tomato, 1 cucumber, 1 carrot, 1 onion slice, 1 slice of tofu, 2 teaspoons of red wine vinegar, 4 pieces of melba toast.

Instructions: Finely chop bell pepper, tomato, cucumber, carrot, onion, and tofu. Add red wine vinegar and serve with melba toast.

Suggested Beverage:
Tangy Banana Pick-Me-Up

Lots of color as well as lots of flavor is the hallmark of this meal. And lots of color means lots of nutrition. The tasty onion helps the control of blood sugar. In addition, a 1960s study determined that consuming onions lowered overall cholesterol even for patients on high fat diets. Bell peppers, whether green, red, orange, yellow or purple, are great sources of beta carotene and Vitamin C. They're also noteworthy for their content of silicon. Its sharp, yet sweet flavor contributes even more to an already tasty dish.

Dinner:

Flounder—Veggie Platter

Ingredients: 4 ounces of broiled filet of flounder, 1 serving of English peas, 1 baked sweet potato, 1 slice whole wheat bread, 1 teaspoon of lemon juice, 1 pat of butter, pepper.

Instructions: Prepare flounder and add lemon juice. Lightly butter bread and sweet potato. Pepper sweet potato. Serve flounder, sweet potato and bread with English peas.

Suggested Beverage:
Blueberry Mash

Fish devotees will take delight in this delicious dish. The flounder, although contributing some fat calories, contains potassium and only a modest amount of sodium. The peas also contain a generous amount of potassium as does the sweet potato. And with the sweet potato, you won't have to worry about your recommended daily allowance of vitamin A. Its content of carotene is so rich, that one medium baked potato will meet, if not exceed the recommended allowance!

Vegetable Deluxe

Ingredients: 1 serving of yellow squash, 1 serving of brown rice, 1 serving of black-eyed peas, 1 serving of broccoli, 1 slice of onion, pepper.

Instructions: Cook squash with onion. Cook rice, peas, and broccoli. Pepper to taste and serve.

Suggested Beverage:
Vinegar Fruit Soda

The onion will give the squash a lively flavor. Of course, the squash is low in fat. It also contains little sodium. The rice contributes fiber as well as a notable amount of protein, and is more nutritious than the white variety. You will also get a good dose of vitamin C from the peas, as well as fiber and potassium. There is also a measure of soluble fiber in broccoli—and broccoli is one of the few calcium-containing vegetables. In fact, the American Cancer Society suggests that broccoli be eaten several times each week.

Chicken on a Veggie Plate

Ingredients: 6 ounces of broiled skinless chicken breast, 1 serving of cooked turnip greens, 1 baked potato, 1 slice whole grain bread, ½ teaspoon apple cider vinegar, 1 pat of butter, paprika.

Instructions: Mix apple cider vinegar with greens. Butter bread and potato. Add a dash of paprika to chicken. Serve with greens, potato, and bread.

Suggested Beverage:
Tropic Delight on the Grapefruit Rocks

Your main source of fat from this meal, of course, is the chicken. But by shedding the skin, the fat grams will be cut almost in half, while the protein, iron, niacin, and zinc content will go largely unaffected. The white meat, such as that of the breast, makes it all the better. It contains less fat grams than its dark meat counterpart but more protein, niacin, potassium, and magnesium—and less sodium!

The greens furnish a huge amount of vitamin A and C as well as a lot of fiber. The potato also contributes a good share of fiber and a great deal of potassium.

Snacks:

• Any fresh fruit, such as apples, grapefruits, and oranges
• Any dried fruit, such as raisins and dates
• Mashed avocado halves with lemon juice and pepper*
• A raw carrot
• A lightly buttered baked potato
• A slice of lightly buttered whole grain bread
• A small serving of unsalted nuts
• Additional servings of any of the suggested drinks
• Decaffeinated tea or coffee

   * Although avocados are high in fat, they are a fruit and that fat content comes largely in the form of the unsaturated variety, not the saturated kind commonly found in considerable quantities in animal products. The big upside: they contain a high amount of protein and fiber.

Extended Diet Summary

By now you get the idea. A diet devoid of all processed snack foods, short on animal products, and long on fruits, vegetables, whole grains, and beans, including the steady use of grapefruit and apple cider vinegar, will work wonders in helping you to shed unwanted pounds.

Any of these meal suggestions can, of course, be varied, but remember it is better to interchange different fruit or vegetable items among themselves rather than to substitute an animal product for a vegetable. You will certainly improve your position more if you swap meats for dairy products. As Dr. Neal Barnard, author of "Foods That Cause You To lose Weight" puts it, "if you are eating meat you are eating someone else's fat and someone else's concentrated stored calories".

Better still, substitute vegetables for animal products (both dairy and meat), since the more items you consume which contain fat, the more you will impede your progress.

Now your diet plan should be firmly in place. Before we begin, however, let's see how we can get the most out of it.

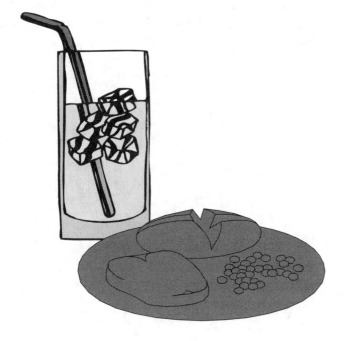

Part 3

On to Victory

Chapter 8

Sound Strategy for a Successful Diet

In order to draw the maximum benefit from your grape-fruit and apple cider vinegar combo diet, it is important to shop wisely, store food properly and prepare it in the best possible way. This will help insure that your body receives the highest amount of nourishment—and an adequately nourished body is not only healthier, it tends to get hungry less often.

Diet-Wise Shopping

You will do well to spend most of your shopping time at the produce counters. That's where you'll, of course, find the most nourishment without the cost of fat.

Make sure to examine all fruits and vegetables carefully. The fresher they are, the longer they will keep and the more nourishment they will retain. Buy canned and frozen vegetables only if absolutely necessary. Even they inevitably lose some nutrition from being processed.

Purchase as many organically grown items as you can. The more pesticide residues you receive from your food, the harder it is on the body. The highest concentration of pesticide residues are generally found in strawberries, bell peppers, spinach, cherries grown in the United States, and peaches. Unknown to many, organic products are 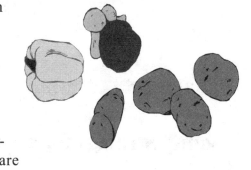 not only pesticide-free, but are grown using natural fertilizers, which give it more nutrition. Organic produce can be more expensive, but don't let that dissuade you. After all, don't you deserve the best?

Minimize your dependence on boxed, packaged foods. They are heavily processed, and have not only lost a lot of their original nutrient content, but often contain preservatives that may create allergies—or worse. In addition, they usually contain refined sugar. Therefore, items that you don't need such as cookies, cupcakes, and chips should be avoided completely—even if they display "low-fat" or "no-fat" on the label. When shopping for items such as cereal, bread, pasta, and yogurt, read the labels carefully. Search for products which at least possess a minimum of preservatives. Look for "low-fat" or "no-fat" on the label on these items. If possible, try to find organic products here, too. And observe all expiration dates. Also, unless you're expecting a blizzard, don't over buy.

It would be far too inefficient to offer specific shopping advice for all the individual grocery items, so in the interest of expediency, here are some helpful shopping tips for the grapefruit and apple cider vinegar:

When shopping for grapefruits, don't be discouraged by the reddish-brown color you often spot on the yellow skin of a grapefruit. This normal occurrence is called "russeting" and it doesn't affect the flavor. However, one should avoid any grapefruits with skin that is rough, wrinkled or ridged. This indicates a thick skin and that means there will be less fruit inside. If grapefruits feel heavy for their size and the skin is thin, not only do you get more fruit, but that fruit should be juicy and flavorful. Also avoid fruit that is soft. It should feel springy—and be flat at both ends.

Try using your nose when selecting grapefruits. A sweet, fragrant scent is a sure sign of quality. If you are not able to detect any aroma, however, that does not necessarily mean the quality is not there. Their fragrance is often absent when they have been kept in a cold environment.

As for apple cider vinegar, many have the impression that vinegar is vinegar. Such is not the case. The most common kind of vinegar on grocery store shelves is distilled. Although it is often used for cooking purposes, just about all the nutrition from the original product has been destroyed by heat from the distilling process. Its label makes no reference to apple or any other fruit. Make sure you purchase the real thing. It possesses a deep, golden yellow color and clearly states "apple cider vinegar" on the label. The best variety is raw and unfiltered. Don't be put off by the residue you see at the bottom. That's only a sign you are getting the pure, unfiltered product. Also search for "organic" on the label.

Storing for Best Nutrition

At home, one should also take care in storing foods. Produce must remain fresh until ready for use. Immediately upon returning from the market, refrigerate all items that require it. The longer they remain at room temperature, the more their nutritional content diminishes. If the temperature is hotter, all the worse. Follow storage instructions on all packaged foodstuffs. Many items not requiring refrigeration should at least be stored in a cool, dry place.

Now here is a quick rundown on how to best store grapefruits and apple cider vinegar:

Grapefruits should, of course, be stored uncut. After being sliced, they begin to lose valuable nutrients at once, especially in the way of vitamin C. Placing them in a fruit bowl at room temperature is perfectly permissible. In fact, this tends to keep them extra juicy and they maintain their full flavor. They will keep for approximately two weeks this way. You can certainly place them in the refrigerator. That way they'll keep even longer—perhaps as long as one month. They are best stored here in the crisper drawer, or at least inside a perforated plastic bag. But to insure the fullest flavor possible, take it out of refrigerator a short time before serving.

As far is apple cider vinegar is concerned, storage is no problem. Just keep it in the pantry. It does not require refrigeration and possesses a long shelf life.

Preparation Tips

Before preparing any meal, you will do well to ask yourself of each serving, "Does it have to be cooked?"

Granted, it would be tough to eat uncooked rice or pasta. But often items which are usually cooked, such a broccoli, carrots, and peas, go well in a raw salad. Its much more easily prepared and more healthful for the stomach. When cooking, stay away from frying. This involves vegetable oils, which possess fat. In addition, fried foods are exposed to too much heat for too long. This breaks down the enzymes and essential fats and then when consumed they tend to create problems such as clogging the blood vessels. Baking and broiling are better. At that, don't cook any longer than necessary and use the lowest temperature practical.

Look for opportunities to substitute apple cider vinegar for another comparable ingredient in recipes, or to merely add it to the recipe. You can also often plug in healthy substitutes for other items. For instance, try using salsa for sugar-laden catsup, honey for refined sugar (not that you'll consider using refined sugar in your diet, will you?) and, of course, apple cider vinegar for salt. Unsalted seasonings are also a good choice.

You might also want to substitute soy milk for cow's milk. It contains all the amino acids necessary to make a complete protein like any animal milk, and it contains the right kind of fat. In fact, when cooking and baking, you can substitute water or any vegetable juice, in recipes calling for milk. If you really want to get innovative, you might even want to try using apple juice as a substitute for milk on cereal.

You can even fashion a light cream for cooking purposes from nuts—yes nuts. Take a half cup of almonds, pine nuts or filberts. Cover them in water and soak overnight. Drain water the next day, place in a blender with enough water to cover them again, then mix into a cream. Add water if necessary to achieve the consistency you desire. This should make about 1 quart.

Now here are some more ideas in which to use grapefruits and apple cider vinegar:

Grapefruit is not only tasty in fruit salads, but also in chicken salads. In many recipes, it can be substituted for oranges—not that oranges are a bad idea. Grapefruits also go well with spicy foods such as chili. They can be used as a poaching liquid for chicken and also in marinades for poultry or fish. As mentioned previously, it is more nutritious when serving grapefruit alone to peel it and serve the individual slices.

As we have already seen, apple cider vinegar can be used in soups and drinks and on salads as a dressing either by itself or mixed with other ingredients such as vegetable oil. It can also, in fact, be added to dips, as well as a number of other recipes. If you dare, apple cider vinegar can even be taken straight from the bottle in a teaspoon!

Now you have all the basic facts. This should give you an extra edge in the bid to reach your weight loss goal. Before we wrap everything up, though, let's consider a practice that should accompany any worthwhile diet—exercise.

Chapter 9

The Beneficial Effects of Exercise

Obviously, what we eat plays a major role in how much we weigh. But exercise cannot be overlooked as a factor. The more activity the body is engaged in, the more calories are burned off. Unfortunately, far too many of us have become button-pushers. Active fingers on TV remotes, computer keyboards, and even automobile dashboards don't burn much fuel.

Calories Burned: A Comparison

On the average, we burn over 200 calories a day less than did those three decades ago.

We seem to frown on exercise as something that's too much work. But we're not talking about boot camp, deep knee calisthenics. Exercise does not have to be, and should not be a burden. In fact, there is a lot of beneficial exercise that can be enjoyable.

Choose something you will enjoy and don't start out by overdoing it. This could result in injury because your body is not yet conditioned or be so demanding that it will discourage you from sticking with it. If you have been inactive for a long time, first try a few simple exercises spanning not more than a few minutes at one stretch, and space them out through the day.

A Caution About Exercise

Those over forty or those who have a history of illness should consult a physician before embarking on an exercise program.

A Walk on the Brisk Side

Walking is the best choice. All you require is a good pair of shoes. It's an easy exercise and for the same distance, a brisk walk actually burns approximately the same number of calories as that of a slow run. Additionally, the more you weigh while walking, the more calories you will burn. For the record, a slow walk for a 120-pound person will consume about three calories per minute; for someone over 200 pounds that figure rises to five. A more brisk pace would render a caloric loss of six and twelve respectively. Most of us should be able to walk at least a half-hour per day. That's the recommended length of time. If you don't want to do it everyday, consider walking an hour three days a week. In fact, that's a better scenario. Exercising the same muscle groups everyday can be counterproductive because that tends to break down the muscle fibers.

You might also consider putting walking into use for an addition purpose. Why not hike down to your local grocery store, if it's not too far away, for that loaf of bread you forgot to pick up the last time you shopped? You'll be burning body fuel, not fuel from the gas tank of your car.

And here are a few more ideas to consider to encourage the habit of walking more. Take the stairs rather than an elevator or escalator. Park your car farther away from shopping mall entrances. Get out of your car when banking, rather than pulling up to the drive-in window.

Other Activities

Other ideas include bicycling, swimming, golf, tennis, and even gardening. Vegetable gardening is especially useful, since it not only provides exercise but eventually fresh produce as well. The activity doesn't necessarily have to be an outside one, but it's always better to get fresh air and sunshine while exercising. Everyone needs a break from the indoor air, which often gets stale from such things as chemicals, molds, and cigarette smoke. And sunlight is important for the body's production of vitamin D.

Some activities will be more effective than others. Walking (especially brisk walking) and cycling fall into this category, as does any exercise that requires continuous, vigorous motion. This increases your heartbeat and leaves you breathing heavily. Activities such as golf and gardening do not offer the same benefit, but are nevertheless helpful to some degree.

Include a friend in your activity and you will be more likely to keep at it—and so, for that matter, will the friend. If boredom sets in, consider expanding your activities. Walk one day and play a round of tennis on another day.

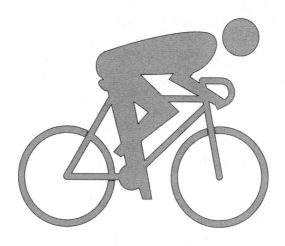

Activities most effective for burning calories include walking and cycling because a continuous, vigorous motion is required.

Activities That Burn Calories

- Walking
- Bicycling
- Swimming
- Golf
- Tennis
- Gardening
- Dancing
- Weight Lifting

- Volleyball
- Rowing
- Bowling
- Running
- Baseball
- Basketball
- Squash
- Handball

More Upside About Exercise

Exercising offers an additional bonus for the weight conscious. The body will continue burning fuel at the same rate for hours afterward. And it also tones muscles. That's important because muscles burn calories and help keep your metabolism high—just what one needs when endeavoring to lose weight. In fact, this actually carries itself one step farther. Since muscles are active to some degree even when one is not exercising, they demand more fuel so your metabolic rate rises. Moreover, they must burn some calories just to continue to exist.

Furthermore, regular exercise will strengthen your heart, lungs, and circulatory system, increase your flexibility and strength, and even improve your psychological state—which in itself could very well help you stick to your eating plans.

Those are the facts. Exercise doesn't have to be difficult or boring and it holds a lot of benefits. It's a perfect addition to your grapefruit and apple cider vinegar combo diet. All you have to do is choose your activity and go for it.

Chapter 10

Success—At Last

You are now armed with all the information you need for your grapefruit and apple cider vinegar combo diet. And you should have the hang of it by now. Rather than imposing a rigid regimen, this book is designed to give you constructive ideas as to what kinds of foods to eat while incorporating grapefruit and apple cider vinegar into your diet.

No matter which diet you choose and no matter how you tailor that diet to suit your taste, remember to remain well within the guidelines. Go heavy on fruits and vegetables and light on animal products. The best scenario is to drop *all* unhealthful fattening foods. You receive all the nourishment you require from fruits, vegetables, whole grains, and beans, along with very little fat. Consume as many raw items as you can to get the full nutritional benefits. Also make sure to get a balance. Regularly eat different kinds of both fruits vegetables. That way you will not neglect full nutrition, while the various flavors and textures will keep your meals appealing. In reality, every time you depart from this, you're altering a perfect formula.

You will likely be tempted to cheat—but remember, the more fattening food you take in the more you will impede your progress. In the end, it's up to you as to how faithful you will remain. Hopefully, this book will not only furnish you with the information you need to begin your grapefruit and apple cider vinegar combo diet, but help you develop better eating habits so the excess weight will stay off.

The bottom line is that if you follow these guidelines, you should see success. That covers the ground. Now it's time to get started. Choose your diet plan and go for it—and good luck.

Appendix A

Producing Homemade Apple Cider Vinegar

For those so inclined, here are instructions for making apple cider vinegar. It's the easiest kind of vinegar to make at home and something that can be fun for the entire family. In addition, it has the advantage of allowing you to adjust the exact flavor to suit your personal taste.

The apples should be fresh, whole fruit and preferably organically produced. Avoid bruised skins and look for fruit that is reasonably firm. Apples that smell especially sweet possess a richer sugar content. This will produce stronger vinegar. Tart fruit, on the other hand, will result in a sharper flavor. Red apples are generally the sweetest, although they might not always be as firm; green ones tend to possess a more tart flavor but are usually crisper. Apples obtained late in the season are best. Any variety will suffice. Just make certain they are ripe. If you don't plan to use them at once, store them in the refrigerator. Their freshness will be preserved longer. Keep in mind, though, that fresh fruit has already lost some of its vitamin value only 24 hours after being picked. The longer the storage time, the more nutrition is lost.

If organic fruit isn't available, wash what you do have thoroughly. This will by no means eliminate all pesticide residues, but it will be of some help. In reality, there will most likely be at least some residual traces of pesticides inside. That's the reason an organic product is so important. Obviously, it's a good idea to wash all fruits and vegetables thoroughly anyway if only to remove any soil bacteria which might be present.

Apple Cider Vinegar Tip

For a more thorough job of washing your fruit, you may want to use apple cider vinegar itself. It's an excellent all-round cleaner.

After the apples have been washed, chop them up and allow them to sit until they begin to turn brown. Next, use a cider press to crush them. The result will be an aromatic brew golden brown in color known as "pomace". Continue to squeeze until liquid begins to flow from the press. You have now created what is called sweet cider. Use a glass container to collect and store it.

At this point it might occur to you that all this squeezing is more trouble than it's worth. "Why not just use apple juice?" you might say. First, apple juice from the store shelf may have undergone pasteurization, and it contains preservatives. Because of this, it will not properly ferment. Second, the juice alone does not contain the peel which itself contains some important nutrients—including the ones that help with weight control.

After the container is filled, it must be capped to keep air away from the cider until it matures. But rather than sealing the top in conventional fashion, use a balloon. As the sugar is converted to alcohol, carbon dioxide is released and the balloon will expand to accommodate it. This initial fermenting process will require several weeks, perhaps as much as eight. The exact time varies according to the sugar content of the cider and the ambient temperature—the optimum temperature being 80 degrees F (26 ½ degrees C). When the balloon ceases to expand, you have completed the creation of hard cider and you're ready for the next step.

Don't allow the recommended temperature to vary too much, however. If it gets too cool, spores prevalent in the air that initiate the fermenting process will become dormant. If it gets too hot, the bacteria required for fermenting will be killed.

Pour the hard cider into a wide-mouthed container. A wooden container is best sense it promotes better fermentation. In addition, it helps the final product taste better. If you notice gray foam resting on top of the cider, don't worry. It is excess yeast, which can easily be skimmed off.

Place a clean cloth securely over the top. You want the cider exposed to the air but you don't want dust and uninvited bugs contaminating it. Store it in a warm dark place and be patient. After several months, you will have created apple cider vinegar.

To hasten the fermenting process, cover the liquid surface with "mother-of-vinegar". It can be purchased at some health food stores. "Mother-of-vinegar" or "mother" for short is the frothy mass found floating on top of a finished batch of cider vinegar. You will notice it when your vinegar has matured. It will prove handy if you plan on making more apple cider vinegar.

**Instructions for Homemade
Apple Cider Vinegar**

- Wash fresh, whole apples
- Chop and allow to sit until brown
- Crush in cider press
- Collect/store the sweet cider which is produced in a glass container
- Cap container with balloon until cider matures (maximum 8 weeks)
- Pour hard cider into wide-mouthed wooden container
- Place clean cloth securely over top
- Store in warm, dark place for several months

Appendix B

Healthful Low-Fat Foods

This appendix has been included to give you an idea of just how much variety we have in healthful, low-fat foods. The combination of vegetable dishes is surprisingly large. Fruits salads can come in many forms. The wide assortment of homemade drinks that can be whipped up from these foods is far more than most probably realize. You can go as far in preparing meals and beverages as your imagination will take you.

Of course, this list is by no means complete. Look it over and see if you can discover items that have been left out.

Healthful, Low-Fat Foods

Acerola
Alfalfa Sprouts
Apple
Apple Cider
    Vinegar
Apricot
Artichokes
Asparagus
Banana
Barley
Beans
Beets
Blueberry
Bok Choy
Broccoli
Brussels Sprouts
Cabbage
Cantaloupe
Carrot
Cauliflower
Celery
Cherry
Corn
Cranberry
Cucumber
Dates
Fennel
Fig

Garlic
Gingerroot
Grapefruit
Grapes
Greens
Honey
Honeydew
    Melon
Jicama
Kale
Kiwi
Leeks
Lemon
Lettuce
Lime
Mango
Millet
Nectarine
Oats
Onion
Orange
Papaya
Parsnips
Pasta
Peach
Pear
Peas
Peppers

Persimmon
Pineapple
Plantain
Plum
Potato
Prunes
Pumpkin
Radish
Raisins
Raspberry
Red Wine
    Vinegar
Rice
Spinach
Squash
Strawberry
Sweet Potato
Swiss Chard
Tangerine
Tomato
Turnips
Watercress
Watermelon
Wheat Germ
Wheat Grass
Yam

Glossary

Acetic Acid: A sour, colorless liquid compound which is found in vinegar.

Adipose Cells: The cells of the adipose tissue, which hold the potential to draw fat from the blood.

Adipose Tissue: A collection a minute cells which draw fat from the blood.

Alpha-linolenic: The fatty acid known as omega-3.

Amino Acids: A group of compounds that serve as units of structure of the proteins.

Ascorbic Acid: Vitamin C.

Beta Carotene: A natural occurring substance in grapefruit and other foods that the human body converts into vitamin A.

Bioflavonoids: A group of approximately 500 compounds that provide color to citrus fruits and vegetables. Along with vitamin C, bioflavonoids help activate the accumulation of fat-freeing hormones and enzymes and boost the benefits of vitamin C as much as twenty times. Sometimes known as vitamin P.

Carbohydrates: Substances that are broken down into simple sugars in the body to be used as fuel. Simple carbohydrates are found in fruit and complex carbohydrates (those with molecules composed of longer, more complex chains) are contained in vegetables and whole grains.

Carotenes: Naturally occurring substances found in fruits and vegetables of which beta carotene is an example.

Cellulose: A kind of fiber that, among other things, moves waste through the colon more rapidly, thereby assisting in the prevention of constipation; found in foods such as apples, broccoli, cabbage, carrots, cucumber skins, and whole wheat flour.

Chromium: A trace mineral essential for keeping blood sugar stable, thereby stopping the craving for the wrong kind of foods.

Citric Acid: An acid derived from citrus fruits.

Coumarins: Substances found in many whole grains, fruits, and vegetables (including grapefruit), which act as natural blood thinners.

Enzymes: Substances produced in plants that help humans digest them.

Fiber: That portion of plant-based foods (fruits, vegetables, whole grains, and nuts) that doesn't digest. It simply pushes its way through your digestive tract, while keeping everything else moving to aid digestion. It contributes texture to the product and a more filling effect is produced. There are different kinds of fiber: pectin, cellulose, lignin, etc. There are also two classes of fiber: soluble, of which pectin is an example and insoluble, of which cellulose is an example.

Galacturonic Acid: A compound found only in grapefruit.

Lignin: A kind of fiber, which, among other things, helps speed food through the stomach; found in plant-based foods such as eggplant, green beans, pears, radishes, and strawberries.

Linoleic: The fatty acid known as omega-6.

Lycopene: A relative of beta carotene found in red grapefruit and other red fruits and vegetables, thought to prevent cancer of the prostate, colon, bladder, cervix, and lung.

Omega-3: An essential fat that helps raise the metabolic rate.

Omega-6: An essential fat that helps prevent adverse effects on the adrenal and the thyroid glands.

Pectin: A soluble fiber found in grapefruit, apples, and other healthy foods.

Peristalsis: The rhythmic, wavelike motion of the walls of certain hollow organs, such as the intestine.

Potassium: A mineral that helps maintain the fluid balance in the body's cells by transporting water to the kidneys to be excreted.

Protein: A substance contained in all vegetable and animal matter that supplies the amino acids, the building blocks of the body.

Saturated fat: An unhealthy kind of fat found chiefly in animal products.

Sodium: A mineral abundantly occurring in nature in compounds—especially common salt; found in its healthy organic form in proper nutritional quantities in vegetables such as celery and spinach.

Terpenes: Compounds existing in plants and animals; helps to protect arteries from disease.

Tofu: A bean curd derived from soy beans; serves as an excellent meat substitute.

Triglycerides: Fat like substances similar to cholesterol found in the blood.

Tryptophan: An essential amino acid found in most proteins in small quantities; important in the synthesis of the vitamin niacin; useful in weight control in that helps prevent the tendency to crave sweets.

Unsaturated fat: A healthy kind of fat found in small quantities in fruits, vegetables, and grains; also found in larger quantities in nuts, seeds, and vegetable oil.

Vitamins: Substances found in most foods and essential for the normal functioning of the body, including the regulation of the metabolism.

Bibliography

Barnard, Neal. Foods that Cause You to Lose Weight: The Negative Calorie Effect. McKinney, Texas: The Magni Group, Inc., 1992.

Bragg, Paul C., Patricia Bragg. Apple Cider Vinegar: Miracle Health System. Santa Barbara, California: Health Science, 1992.

Bragg, Paul C., Patricia Bragg. Bragg Healthy Lifestyle: Vital Living to 120! Santa Barbara, California: Health Science, 1992.

Davis, Karen. Nature's Healing Foods. Boca Raton, Florida: Globe Communications Corp., 1995.

Evans, William J. Biomarkers: The Keys to Lifelong Vitality. Bottom Line Tomorrow. Volume 5 Number 11. November, 1997.

Hausman, Patricia, Judith Benn Hurley. The Healing Foods: The Ultimate Authority on the Curative Power of Nutrition. Emmaus, Pennsylvania: Rodale, 1989.

Jarvis, D. C. Folk Medicine: A New England Almanac of Natural Health Care from a Noted Vermont Country Doctor. New York, New York: Fawcett Crest, 1982.

Kordich, Jay. The Juiceman's Power of Juicing. New York, New York: William Morrow and Company, Inc., 1992.

Mindell, Earl L. Amazing Apple Cider Vinegar. New Canaan, Connecticut: Keats Publishing, Inc., 1996.

Mindell, Earl L. Earl Mindell's Anti-Aging Bible. New York, New York: Simon & Schuster, 1996.

Mirkin, Gabe, M. D. The 20/30 Fat & Fiber Diet Plan. New York, New York: Harper Collins Publishers, 1998.

Oberbeil, Klaus. Lose Weight with Apple Vinegar. McKinney, Texas: The Magni Group, Inc., 1999.

Quillin, Patrick. Honey, Garlic & Vinegar: Home Remedies and Recipes. North Canton, Ohio: The Leader Co., Inc., 1996.

Ross, Julia, M. A. The Diet Cure. New York, New York: Viking, 1999.

Scott, Cyril, John Lust. Cider Vinegar. New York, New York: Benedict Lust Publications, 1992.

Thacker, Emily. The Vinegar Book. Canton, Ohio: Tresco Publishers, 1996.

Thacker, Emily. The Vinegar Diet. Canton, Ohio: Tresco Publishers, 1997.

Index